Ketogenic and Intermittent Fasting Diet

I0145964

A New Complete Diet Guide for Vegetarians, with Intermittent Fasting Strategy, to lose weight and Fast Fat Burning. With delicious recipes for snacks and desserts.

Sebi Alan Guntry

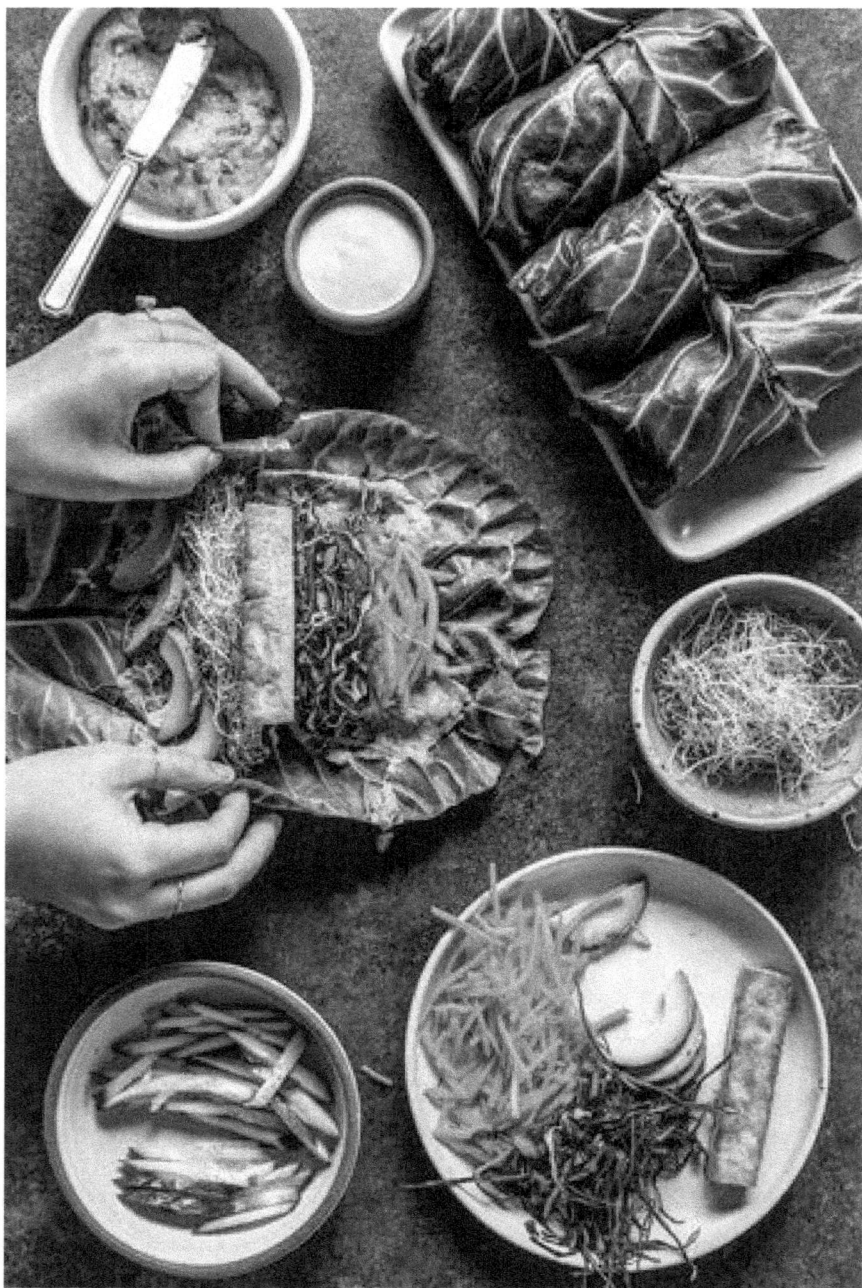

Tables of contains

Introduction

A keto diet for vegetarians is focused on proportionately eating more foods primarily from plants and cutting back on animal-derived foods. However, it does not necessarily involve eliminating entire food groups and lean sources of protein. This means, those on a plant-based diet may still opt to eat some meat.

Going vegan, on the other hand, means being strictly against animal products in any form—from never eating meat and dairy products to not patronizing products tested on animals and not wearing animal products such as leather.

A healthy keto plant-based diet generally emphasizes meeting your nutritional needs by eating more whole plant foods, while reducing the intake of animal products. Whole foods refer to natural, unrefined or minimally refined foods. Plant foods consist of those that do not have animal ingredients such as meat, eggs, honey, milk and other dairy products.

In contrast, those on a vegetarian diet may still eat processed and refined foods. Vegetarians can even eat fast foods, junk food and other salty snacks guilt-free.

Once you get started with this diet, you will notice a huge difference in how you feel each day. From the time that you wake up in the morning, you will feel that you have more energy, and that you do not get tired as easily as before. You will also have more mental focus and fewer mood-related problems.

As for digestion, a plant-based diet is also said to improve how the digestive system works. In fact, dieters confirm fewer incidences of stomach pains, bloating, indigestion and hyperacidity.

Then there's the weight loss benefit that we cannot forget about. Since a keto plant-based diet means eating fruits, vegetables, and whole grains that have fewer calories and are lower in fat, you will enjoy weight loss benefits that some other fad diets are not able to provide.

Aside from helping you lose weight; it maintains ideal weight longer because this diet is easier to sustain and does not require elimination of certain food groups.

Don't worry about not getting enough nutrients from your food intake. This diet provides all the necessary nutrients including proteins, vitamins, minerals, carbohydrates, fats, and antioxidants. And again, that's because it does not eliminate any food group but only encourages you to focus more on keto plant-based food products.

As you can imagine, humans have been consuming a keto plant-based diet before the invention of McDonald's and some of our other favorite fast-food chains. To begin our journey, I am going to start us off in the times of the hunter-gatherer. While we could go back even further (think Ancient Egypt!), I believe this is where a keto plant-based diet becomes most relevant.

The hunter-gatherer time period is where we find the earliest evidence of hunting. While we do have a long history of eating meat, this was a point in time where consuming meat was very limited. Of course, humans eating meat does not mean we were carnivores; in fact, the way we are built tells us differently. Yes, we can consume meat, but humans are considered omnivores. You can tell this from our jaw design, running speeds, alimentary tract, and the fact we don't have claws attached to our fingers. History also tells us we are omnivores by nature; however, the evolution of our human brains led us to become hunters so that we could survive.

The need for hunting did not come around until our ancestors left tropical regions. Other locations influenced the availability of keto plant-based foods. Instead of enduring winter with limited amounts of food, we had to adapt! Of course, out of hunger, animal-flesh becomes much more appealing. This early in time, our ancestors did not have a grocery store to just pop in and buy whatever they needed. Instead, they used the opportunity of hunting and gathering to keep themselves alive.

Eventually, we moved away from hunting and gathering and started to become farmers. While this timeline is a bit tricky and agricultural history began at different points in different parts of the world, all that matters is that at some point; animals started to become domesticated and dairy, eggs, and meat all became readily available. Once this started, humans no longer needed to hunt nor gather because the farmers provided everything we could desire

While starting a keto plant-based diet is an excellent idea and has many wonderful benefits let's be honest, you are mostly here to benefit yourself. It is fantastic that you are deciding to put you and your health first. You deserve to be the best version of yourself, with a little bit of legwork, you will be there in no time

To some people, a keto plant-based diet is just another fad diet. There are so many diets on the market right now, why is plant-based any different? Whether you are looking to lose weight, reverse disease, or just love animals.

A plant-based diet is so much more than just eating fruits and vegetables. This is a lifestyle where you are encouraged to journey to a better version of yourself. As you improve your eating habits, you will need something to do with all of your new found energy! It is time to gain control over your eating habits and figure out how food truly does affect our daily lives! Below, you will find the amazing benefits a plant-based diet has to offer you.

The Circadian Cycle

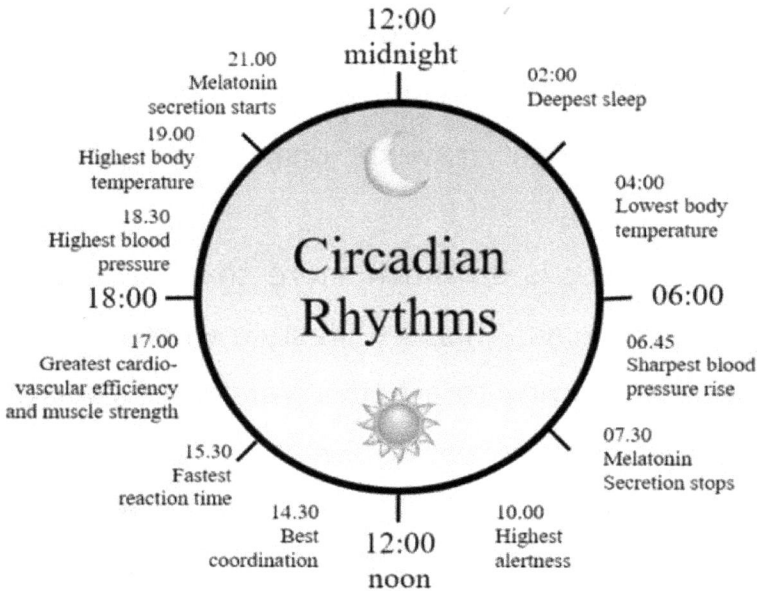

The circadian cycle is nothing more than the set of variations to which our biological activities are subjected on a daily basis:

- Blood pressure
- Body temperature
- Muscle tone
- Heart rate

- Sleep-wake rhythm
- Lipid metabolism

It is of fundamental importance to know our circadian rhythm because depending on the phases of our body needs certain foods and not others.

Foods according to the phases of the cycle:

- between 7 a.m. - 3 p.m. it would be better to take carbohydrates
- between 3 pm and 8 pm is the protein phase

Snacks For Morning And Afternoon

Strawberry Mango Shave Ice

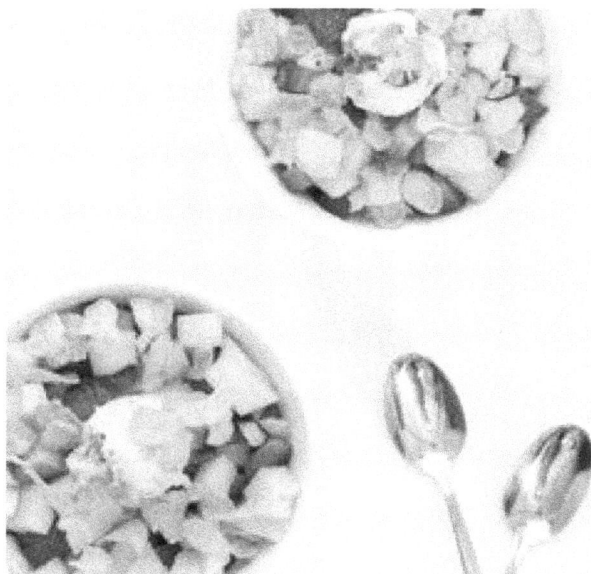

Preparation time: 20 minutes

Cooking time: 10 minutes

Serving: 4

Ingredients:

½ cup superfine sugar, divided

1-cup strawberries, diced

2 diced mangos

2 cups mango juice

½ cup coconut, toasted

Directions:

Add 1 cup water and ¾ cup sugar to a pot and boil over medium heat.

Once boiled, remove from heat and add 2 more cups of water.

Freeze this mixture stirring after every 45 minutes.

Take a blender and add all remaining ingredients and blend until smooth.

Strain the mixture into a container with a pour spout.

For serving, divide the ice into glasses and pour juice and mixture over them.

Serve and enjoy.

Nutrition:

Calories 366

Fat 5.5 g,

Carbs 82.4 g,

Protein 2.7 g

Banana Muffins

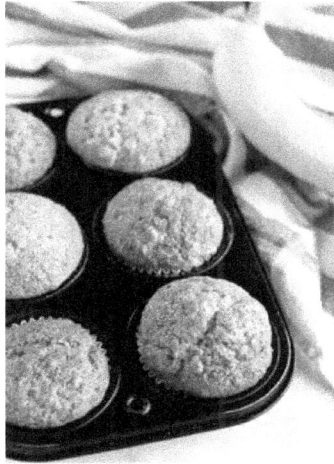

Preparation time: 10 minutes

Cooking time: 15 minutes

Serving: 6

Ingredients:

- 1 cup rolled oats
- 1 medium banana
- 2 tablespoons ground flaxseed
- 1/4 teaspoon sea salt
- 3/4 teaspoon baking powder
- 1/4 teaspoon baking soda
- 3 tablespoons vanilla protein powder
- 1/2 teaspoon vanilla extract. unsweetened
- 2 tablespoons maple syrup

- 5 tablespoons water
- 2/3 cup soy yogurt, unsweetened

Directions:

1. Prepare the flax egg and for this, take a large bowl, place ground flaxseed, stir in water and let it stand for 5 minutes until thickened.
2. Switch on the oven, then set it to 400 degrees F and let it preheat.
3. After 5 minutes, add remaining ingredients into the flax egg and then mix with an electric mixer until incorporated and smooth batter comes together.
4. Take five silicone muffin cups, fill them evenly with batter and then bake for 15 minutes until golden brown.
5. When done, let muffins cool for 10 minutes on a wire rack and then serve.

Nutrition

- Calories 398
- Fat 3.8g
- Carbs 44.2g
- Protein 15g

Chocolate Protein Power Bars

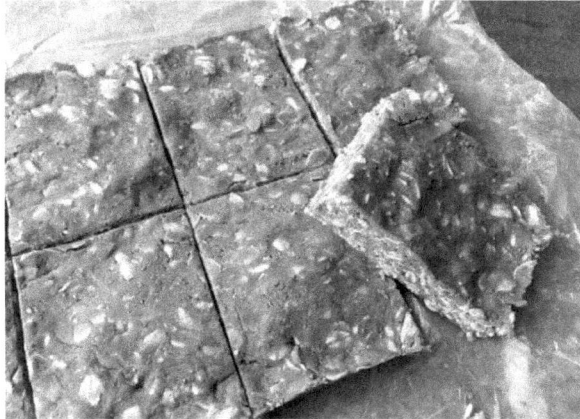

Preparation time: 3 hours

Cooking time: 40 minutes

Serving: 6

Ingredients:

For the Filling:

- 2 cups of quick oats
- 8 Medjool dates pitted
- ¼ teaspoon salt

3½ tablespoons chocolate protein powder

1 teaspoon vanilla extract, unsweetened

2 tablespoons maple syrup

½ teaspoon almond extract, unsweetened

¼ cup of water

For the Coating:

¼ teaspoon almond extract, unsweetened

1¼ cups melted dark chocolate

1 tablespoon coconut oil

Directions:

Prepare the filling and for this, place all of its ingredients in a food processor and then pulse for 2 minutes until well incorporated.

Take a rectangular container, about 3 by 5 inches, place filling in it, then spread it evenly and freeze for a minimum of 3 hours until firm.

Along with the filling, take a small metal tray, line it with parchment paper, and let it chill in the freezer until required.

When ready to coat, take a shallow dish, place

melted chocolate in it, add dark chocolate and coconut oil and then stir until mixed.

Then remove the filling container from the container, transfer the filling block onto a cutting board, and cut it into six squares.

Working on one square at a time, dip it into melted chocolate, wipe the excess chocolate, place it on the chilled metal tray and repeat with the remaining square.

Return the metal tray into the freezer for 30 minutes until chocolate is hard and then serve.

Nutrition

Calories 398

Fat 4.8g

Carbs 49g

Protein 5g

Cherry and Berry Parfait

Preparation time: 8 hours

Cooking time: 5 minutes

Serving: 2

Ingredients:

- 1 cup granola
- 1/4 cup chia seeds
- 1 1/2 cup mixed berries
- 2 tablespoons honey
- 2 teaspoons vanilla extract, unsweetened
- 1 cup almond milk, unsweetened

Directions:

1. Take a large bowl, place chia seeds in it, add honey and vanilla, pour in milk, stir until combined and let it stand in the refrigerator overnight.
2. When ready to eat, stir the chia mixture, divide it evenly between two bowls, top it evenly with mixed berries and granola and then serve.

Nutrition

Calories; 21g

Fat; 4.7g

Carbs; 44.2g

Protein; 0

.5g Sugars

Brownie Batter Bites

Preparation time: 10 minutes

Cooking time: 5 minutes

Serving: 5

Ingredients:

10 tablespoons cocoa powder

4 tablespoons chocolate chips

1/4 teaspoon sea salt

2 teaspoons vanilla extract, unsweetened

6 tablespoons maple syrup

1/4 cup pea protein powder

1/4 cup almond butter

Directions:

Take a large bowl, add all the ingredients in it except for chocolate chips and then stir until well mixed.

Fold in chocolate chips, and then shape the mixture into ten balls, each about 2-inch in size.

Serve straight away.

Nutrition

Calories 248

Fat; 4.7g

Carbs; 44.2g

Protein; 0

.5g Sugars

Chocolate Chia Protein Pudding

Preparation time: 10 minutes

Cooking time: 30 minutes

Serving: 2

Ingredients:

4 tablespoons chia seeds

2 tablespoons vegan chocolate protein powder

2 tablespoons cocoa powder

1 tablespoon maple syrup

1 1/2 cup almond milk, unsweetened

Directions:

Place chia seeds in a food processor, add almond milk and then pulse for 30 seconds until blended.

Add remaining ingredients and then pulse for 1 minute until very smooth.

Distribute the pudding evenly between two bowls, chill in the refrigerator for a minimum of 1 hour and then serve.

Nutrition:

- Calories 298
- Fat; 4.7g
- Carbs; 44.2g
- Protein 33 g

Chocolate Tofu Pudding

Preparation time: 1 hour

Cooking time: 20 minutes

Serving: 4

Ingredients

- 16 ounces silken tofu
- 1 tablespoon instant coffee
- 1/3 cup cacao powder
- 1/4 cup maple syrup
- 2 teaspoons vanilla extract, unsweetened

Directions

Place all the ingredients in the food processor in the order and then pulse at a high setting for 2 minutes until combined and very smooth.

Distribute the pudding among four bowls, chill in the refrigerator for a minimum of 1 hour and then serve.

Nutrition:

Calories 99

Fat; 4g

Carbs; 4g

Protein 50g

Chocolate Mousse

Preparation time: 1 hour

Cooking time: 0 minutes

Serving: 4

Ingredients

- 14 ounces silken tofu
- 1/2 cup chocolate, melted
- 2 tablespoons cacao powder, unsweetened
- 1/8 teaspoon salt
- 1/4 teaspoon ground cinnamon
- 4 tablespoons maple syrup
- 1/2 teaspoon vanilla extract, unsweetened
- 1/4 cup coconut cream

Directions:

Place all the ingredients in the food processor in the order and then pulse at a high setting for 2 minutes until combined and very smooth.

Distribute the mousse among four bowls, chill in the refrigerator for a minimum of 1 hour and then serve.

Nutrition:

Calories 98

Fat 4.7g

Carbs 4.2g

Protein 22 g

Sugars 2

Chocolate Black Bean and Orange Mousse

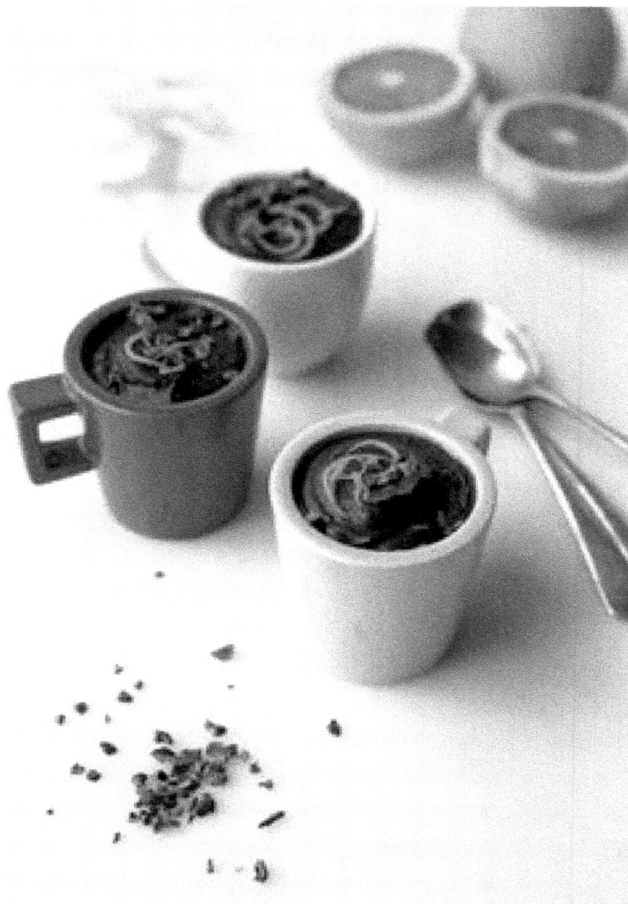

Preparation time: 1 hour

Cooking time: 5 minutes

Serving: 6

Ingredients:

- 15-ounce cooked black beans
- 1 orange, zested
- 1.7 ounces pitted dates
- 5 tablespoons cacao powder, unsweetened
- 1 teaspoon cacao nibs and more for topping
- 8 tablespoons maple syrup
- 2 tablespoons coconut oil, melted
- 4 tablespoons almond milk, unsweetened

Directions:

1. Place dates and black beans in a food processor and then pulse at a high setting for 1 minute.
2. Add remaining ingredients except for orange zest and pulse for 1 minute until blended.
3. Transfer the mousse into a bowl, add orange zest, and then stir until mixed.
4. Distribute the mousse among six bowls, sprinkle some more cacao nibs on top, and then chill in the refrigerator for a minimum of 1 hour.
5. Serve straight away.

Nutrition:

- Calories: 156
- Fat: 8.01g
- Carbohydrate: 20.33g
- Protein: 1.98g
- Sugar: 0.33g
- Cholesterol: 0mg

Carrot Cake Bites

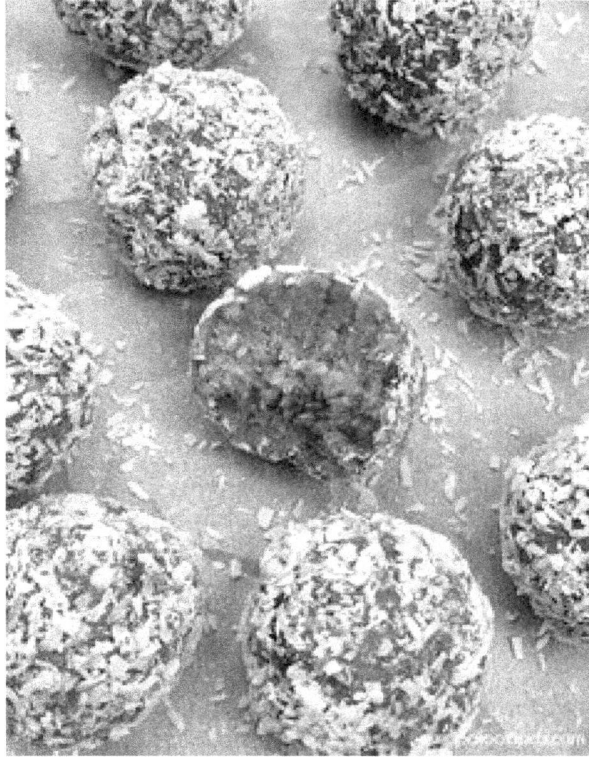

Preparation time: 10 minutes

Cooking time: 0 minutes

Serving: 8

Ingredients:

1 cup chopped carrots

1 cup rolled oats

1/2 cup pecans

1/2 cup Medjool dates

1/2 teaspoon ground nutmeg

1 1/2 teaspoons ground cinnamon

1/4 cup cashew butter

1/2 cup coconut flakes

1/3 cup shredded coconut

Directions:

Place carrots in a food processor, then pulse for 2 minutes until finely chopped and transfer carrots into a large bowl.

Add coconut and pecans into the food processor, pulse for 1 minute until mixture resembles sand, then add dates and oats and blend for another mixture.

Add remaining ingredients except for coconut and then pulse for 2 minutes until the dough comes together.

Shape the dough into small balls, about 1 tablespoon of dough per ball, and then roll the balls into coconut until evenly coated.

Serve straight away.

Nutrition

    Calories: 96

    Fat: 8.8g

    Carbohydrates: 5.12g

    Protein: 1.2g

    Sugar: 0.4g

    Cholesterol: 0mg

Almond Milk

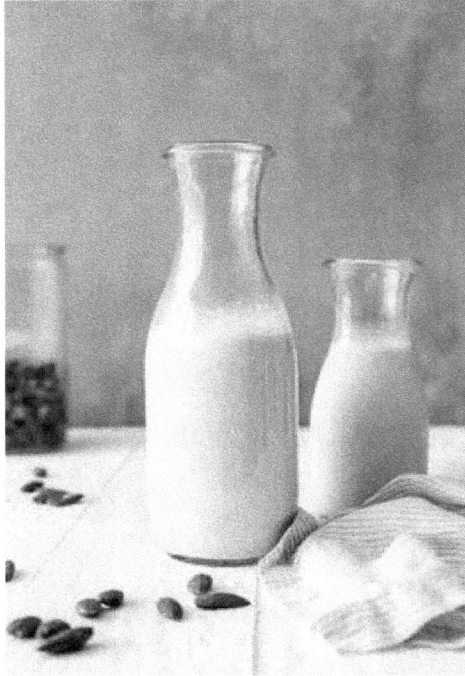

Preparation Time: 10-20 minutes

Cooking Time: 20 minutes plus overnight soaking

Servings: 500ml

Ingredients:

- Blanched almonds: 250g
- Maple syrup: 1 tsp
- Water: 500 ml

Directions:

Soaked almonds in the water overnight

Add maple syrup, blanched almonds, and water to the blender and blend till smoothen

Strain and discard the puree

Shake before serving

Nutrition:

Carbs: 1.3g

Protein: 1.4g

Fats: 2.9g

Calories: 35Kcal

Almond Roasted Veggies Salad

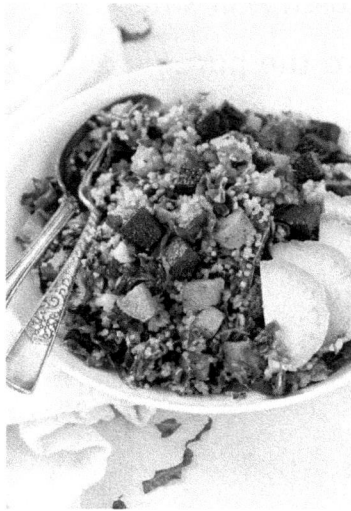

Preparation Time: 10-20 minutes

Cooking Time: 30 minutes

Servings: 4

Ingredients:

- Carrots: 1 cup sliced
- Broccoli: 1 cup sliced
- Cauliflower: 1 cup sliced
- Olive oil: 1 tbsp
- Salt: as per your taste
- Pepper: as per your taste

- Almonds: 1 cup whole roasted
- For the Dressing:
- Lemon: 2 zest and juice
- Mirin: 2 tbsp
- Garlic: 1 clove crushed
- Extra-virgin olive oil: 2 tbsp
- Salt: as per your need

Directions:

1. Add all the vegetables to the baking tray, sprinkle salt and pepper, brush with olive oil and bake for 20 minutes
2. Prepare the dressing by adding all the Ingredients: except oil and combine it slowly at the end whisking to gain the correct consistency
3. Add vegetables to the tray and pour dressing and almonds from the top and serve

Nutrition:

- Carbs: 11g
- Protein: 9.7g
- Fats: 25g

- Calories: 309Kcal

Apple Almond Mix

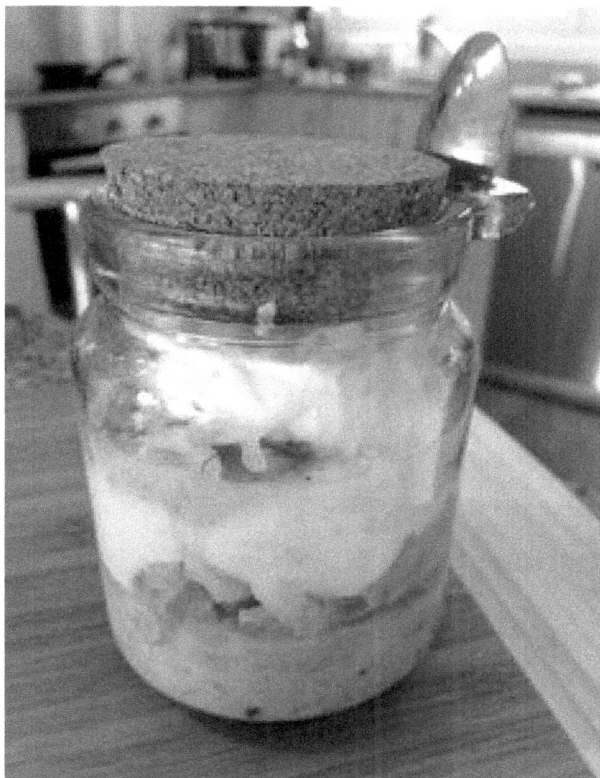

Preparation Time: 10-20 minutes

Cooking Time: 5 minutes

Servings: 4

Ingredients:

- Apple: 4 peeled and diced into bite-sized chunks
- Almond: 1 cup grated

- Lime: 1 juiced
- Sea salt: ½ tsp
- Coconut yogurt to serve

Directions:

- Place all the Ingredients: in a large bowl and shake them well
- Now serve it with some coconut yogurt if you desire

Nutrition:

- Carbs: 31g
- Protein: 7.5g
- Fats: 18.3g
- Calories: 395Kcal

Asian Cabbage Pickle

Preparation Time: 10-20 minutes

Cooking Time: 20 minutes plus marinating

Servings: 6

Ingredients:

- Red cabbage: 1 small
- Ginger: 4cm piece shredded
- Bird's-eye chilies: 2
- Caster sugar: 50g
- Vinegar: 100ml
- Sesame oil: 2 tsp
- Black sesame seeds: 2 tsp

Directions:

1. Take a cabbage
2. Remove the sagging outer leaves and quarter the cabbage
3. Remove the core and put the remaining in a bowl along with ginger and some slit chilies

4. Dissolved the sugar in the mixture of vinegar and sugar then pour 100 ml of water along with 1 teaspoon of salt
5. Marinate the cabbage for 2 hours
6. Take a bowl, drain the cabbage well and pour some sesame seeds and oil

Nutrition:

- Carbs: 5.9g
- Protein: 1.6g
- Fats: 1.7g
- Calories: 53Kcal

Avocado Chaat

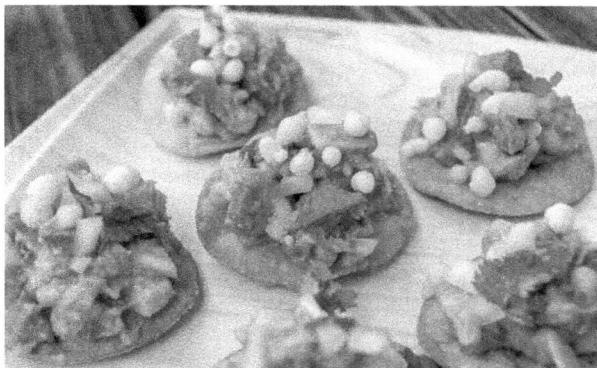

Preparation Time: 10-20 minutes

Cooking Time: 5 minutes

Servings: 4

Ingredients:

- Avocado: 4 peeled and diced into bite-sized chunks
- Chaat masala: 2 tsp
- Lime: 1 juiced
- Sea salt: ½ tsp
- Coconut yogurt to serve

Directions:

Place all the Ingredients: in a large bowl and shake

them well

Now serve it with some coconut yogurt if you desire

Nutrition:

- Carbs:12 g
- Protein: 2.9g
- Fats: 21g
- Calories: 234Kcal

Avocado Potstickers

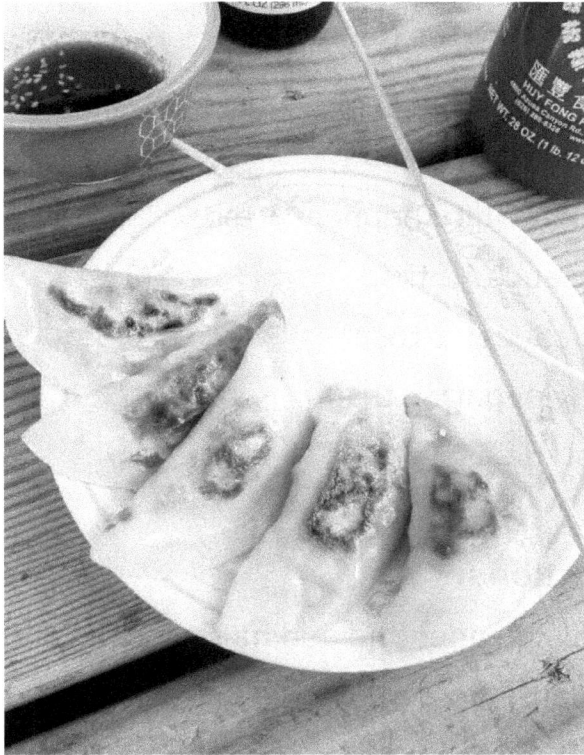

Preparation Time: 10-20 minutes

Cooking Time: 55 minutes

Servings: 36 potstickers

Ingredients:

Edamame: 1lb cooked (shelled)

Ripe avocado: 1 half reserved and one chopped

Bok choy: 1 small stem and leaves separated and diced

Ginger: 1 gm minced

Circle-shaped wonton wrappers: about 36 sheets

Garlic:3 cloves minced

Coconut sugar: 1½ tbsp

Scallions: 1 sliced

Ground white pepper:¼ tsp

Soy sauce: 2 tbsp

Chili sauce: 1 tbsp

Rice vinegar:½ tbsp

Toasted sesame oil: ½ tbsp

Directions:

Take a blender and add half avocado and three quarters of edamame and blend

Give them smooth consistency

Add the mixture to the bowl and add the remaining edamame, avocado, bok choy, green onions, garlic, ginger, and seasonings

Mix them all well

Line the baking sheet with parchment paper and place and wonton wrappers

Add the filling in the middle of the wrapper

Wet the wrapper corner and fold using fingers and do it

will all the wrappers

Bake till golden brown

Nutrition:

- Carbs: 18 g
- Protein: 7 g
- Fats: 3 g
- Calories: 123 Kcal

Avocado Peanut Salad

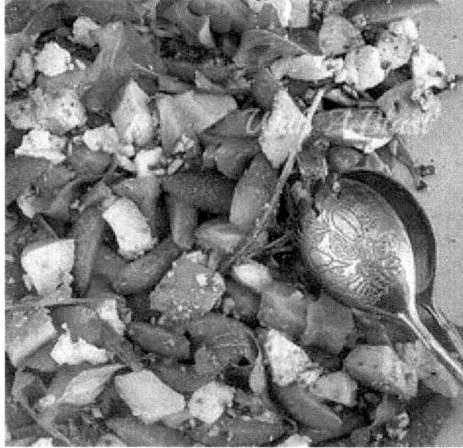

Preparation Time: 10-20 minutes

Cooking Time: 30 minutes

Servings: 4

Ingredients:

- Avocado: 2 cups diced
- Peanuts: ½ cup
- Lemon juice: 1 tbsp
- Mint: ¼ cup leaves torn
- For the Dressing:
- Vinegar: 2 tsp
- Garlic: 1 clove crushed

- Extra-virgin olive oil: 3 tbsp
- Tahini: 2 tbsp
- Lemon: 1 zest and juice
- Salt: as per your need

Directions:

1. Take a pan and add peanuts to roast them dry and crush using hand
2. Prepare the dressing by adding all the Ingredients: except oil and combine it slowly at the end whisking to gain the correct consistency
3. Add avocado to the serving tray
4. Top with peanuts
5. Sprinkle mint leaves and pour lemon juice and serve

Nutrition:

- Carbs: 11.4g
- Protein: 5.7g
- Fats: 34g
- Calories: 379Kcal

Desserts

Key Lime Pie

Preparation Time: 3 hours and 15 minutes

Cooking Time: 0 minute

Servings: 12

Ingredients:

For the Crust:

- ¾ cup coconut flakes, unsweetened
- 1 cup dates, soaked in warm water for 10 minutes in water, drained
- *For the Filling*:
- ¾ cup of coconut meat
- 1 ½ avocado, peeled, pitted
- 2 tablespoons key lime juice
- ¼ cup agave
-

Directions:

Prepare the crust, and for this, place all its ingredients in a food processor and pulse for 3 to 5 minutes until the thick paste comes together.

Take an 8-inch pie pan, grease it with oil, pour crust mixture in it and spread and press the mixture evenly in the bottom and along the sides, and freeze until required.

Prepare the filling and for this, place all its ingredients in a food processor, and pulse for 2 minutes until smooth.

Pour the filling into prepared pan, smooth the top, and freeze for 3 hours until set.

Cut pie into slices and then serve.

Nutrition:

Calories: 213 Cal

Fat: 10 g

Carbs: 29 g

Protein: 1200 g

Fiber: 6 g

Chocolate Mint Grasshopper Pie

Preparation Time: 4 hours and 15 minutes

Cooking Time: 0 minute

Servings: 4

Ingredients:

For the Crust:

- 1 cup dates, soaked in warm water for 10 minutes in water, drained
- 1/8 teaspoons salt
- 1/2 cup pecans
- 1 teaspoons cinnamon
- 1/2 cup walnuts

For the Filling:

- ½ cup mint leaves
- 2 cups of cashews, soaked in warm water for 10 minutes in water, drained
- 2 tablespoons coconut oil
- 1/4 cup and 2 tablespoons of agave
- 1/4 teaspoons spirulina

- 1/4 cup water

Directions:

1. Prepare the crust, and for this, place all its ingredients in a food processor and pulse for 3 to 5 minutes until the thick paste comes together.

2. Take a 6-inch springform pan, grease it with oil, place crust mixture in it and spread and press the mixture evenly in the bottom and along the sides, and freeze until required.

3. Prepare the filling and for this, place all its ingredients in a food processor, and pulse for 2 minutes until smooth.

4. Pour the filling into prepared pan, smooth the top, and freeze for 4 hours until set.

5. Cut pie into slices and then serve.

Nutrition:

- Calories: 223.7 Cal
- Fat: 7.5 g
- Carbs: 36 g
- Protein: 2.5 g
- Fiber: 1 g

Peanut Butter Energy Bars

Preparation Time: 5 hours and 15 minutes

Cooking Time: 5 minutes

Servings: 16

Ingredients:

- 1/2 cup cranberries
- 12 Medjool dates, pitted
- 1 cup roasted almond
- 1 tablespoon chia seeds
- 1 1/2 cups oats
- 1/8 teaspoon salt
- 1/4 cup and 1 tablespoon agave nectar
- 1/2 teaspoon vanilla extract, unsweetened
- 1/3 cup and 1 tablespoon peanut butter, unsalted
- 2 tablespoons water

Directions:

1. Place an almond in a food processor, pulse until chopped, and then transfer into a large bowl.
2. Add dates into the food processor along with oats, pour in water, and pulse for dates are chopped.

3. Add dates mixture into the almond mixture, add chia seeds and berries and stir until mixed.
4. Take a saucepan, place it over medium heat, add remaining butter and remaining ingredients, stir and cook for 5 minutes until mixture reaches to a liquid consistency.
5. Pour the butter mixture over date mixture, and then stir until well combined.
6. Take an 8 by 8 inches baking tray, line it with parchment sheet, add date mixture in it, spread and press it evenly and refrigerate for 5 hours.
7. Cut it into sixteen bars and serve.

Nutrition:
- Calories: 187 Cal
- Fat: 7.5 g
- Carbs: 27.2 g
- Protein: 4.7 g
- Fiber: 2 g

Black Bean Brownie Pops

Preparation Time: 45 minutes

Cooking Time: 2 minutes

Servings: 12

Ingredients:

- 3/4 cup chocolate chips
- 15 ounce cooked black beans
- 1 tablespoon maple syrup
- 5 tablespoons cacao powder
- 1/8 teaspoon sea salt
- 2 tablespoons sunflower seed butter

Directions:

1. Place black beans in a food processor, add remaining ingredients, except for chocolate, and pulse for 2 minutes until combined and the dough starts to come together.
2. Shape the dough into twelve balls, arrange them on a baking sheet lined with parchment paper, then insert a toothpick into each ball and refrigerate for 20 minutes.

3. Then meat chocolate in the microwave for 2 minutes, and dip brownie pops in it until covered.
4. Return the pops into the refrigerator for 10 minutes until set and then serve.

Nutrition:
- Calories: 130 Cal
- Fat: 6 g
- Carbs: 17 g
- Protein: 4 g
- Fiber: 1 g

Lemon Cashew Tart

Preparation Time: 3 hours and 15 minutes

Cooking Time: 0 minute

Servings: 12

Ingredients:

For the Crust:

- 1 cup almonds
- 4 dates, pitted, soaked in warm water for 10 minutes in water, drained
- 1/8 teaspoon crystal salt
- 1 teaspoon vanilla extract, unsweetened

For the Cream:

- 1 cup cashews, soaked in warm water for 10 minutes in water, drained
- 1/4 cup water
- 1/4 cup coconut nectar
- 1 teaspoon coconut oil
- 1 teaspoon vanilla extract, unsweetened
- 1 lemon, Juiced
- 1/8 teaspoon crystal salt
- For the Topping:
- Shredded coconut as needed

Directions:

Prepare the cream and for this, place all its ingredients in a food processor, pulse for 2 minutes until smooth, and then refrigerate for 1 hour.

Then prepare the crust, and for this, place all its ingredients in a food processor and pulse for 3 to 5 minutes until the thick paste comes together.

Take a tart pan, grease it with oil, place crust mixture in it and spread and press the mixture evenly in the bottom and along the sides, and freeze until required.

Pour the filling into the prepared tart, smooth the top, and refrigerate for 2 hours until set.

Cut tart into slices and then serve.

Nutrition:

Calories: 166 Cal

Fat: 10 g

Carbs: 15 g

Protein: 5 g

Fiber: 1 g

Peppermint Oreos

Preparation Time: 2 hours

Cooking Time: 0 minute

Servings: 12

Ingredients:

For the Cookies:

1 cup dates

2/3 cup brazil nuts

3 tablespoons carob powder

2/3 cup almonds

1/8 teaspoon sea salt

3 tablespoons water

For the Crème:

2 tablespoons almond butter

1 cup coconut chips

2 tablespoons melted coconut oil

1 cup coconut shreds

3 drops of peppermint oil

1/2 teaspoon vanilla powder

For the Dark Chocolate:

3/4 cup cacao powder

1/2 cup date paste

1/3 cup coconut oil, melted

Directions:

Prepare the cookies, and for this, place all its ingredients in a food processor and pulse for 3 to 5 minutes until the dough comes together.

Then place the dough between two parchment sheets, roll the dough, then cut out twenty-four cookies of the desired shape and freeze until solid.

Prepare the crème, and for this, place all its ingredients in a food processor and pulse for 2 minutes until smooth.

When cookies have hardened, sandwich crème in between the cookies by placing dollops on top of a cookie and then pressing it with another cookie.

Freeze the cookies for 30 minutes and in the meantime, prepare chocolate and for this, place all its ingredients in a bowl and whisk until combined.

Dip frouncesen cookie sandwich into chocolate, at least two times, and then freeze for another 30 minutes until chocolate has hardened.

Serve straight away.

Nutrition:

Calories: 470 Cal

Fat: 32 g

Carbs: 51 g

Protein: 7 g

Fiber: 12 g

Snickers Pie

Preparation Time: 4 hours

Cooking Time: 0 minute

Servings: 16

Ingredients:

For the Crust:

- 12 Medjool dates, pitted
- 1 cup dried coconut, unsweetened
- 5 tablespoons cocoa powder
- 1/2 teaspoon sea salt
- 1 teaspoon vanilla extract, unsweetened
- 1 cup almonds

For the Caramel Layer:

- 10 Medjool dates, pitted, soaked for 10 minutes in warm water, drained
- 2 teaspoons vanilla extract, unsweetened
- 3 teaspoons coconut oil
- 3 tablespoons almond butter, unsalted
- *For the Peanut Butter Mousse:*
- 3/4 cup peanut butter

- 2 tablespoons maple syrup
- 1/2 teaspoon vanilla extract, unsweetened
- 1/8 teaspoon sea salt
- 28 ounces coconut milk, chilled

Directions:

1. Prepare the crust, and for this, place all its ingredients in a food processor and pulse for 3 to 5 minutes until the thick paste comes together.
2. Take a baking pan, line it with parchment paper, place crust mixture in it and spread and press the mixture evenly in the bottom, and freeze until required.
3. Prepare the caramel layer, and for this, place all its ingredients in a food processor and pulse for 2 minutes until smooth.
4. Pour the caramel on top of the prepared crust, smooth the top and freeze for 30 minutes until set.
5. Prepare the mousse and for this, separate coconut milk and its solid, then add solid from coconut milk into a food processor, add remaining ingredients and then pulse for 1 minute until smooth.

6. Top prepared mousse over caramel layer, and then freeze for 3 hours until set.
7. Serve straight away.

Nutrition:

- Calories: 456 Cal
- Fat: 33 g
- Carbs: 37 g
- Protein: 8.3 g
- Fiber: 5 g

Double Chocolate Orange Cheesecake

Preparation Time: 4 hours

Cooking Time: 0 minute

Servings: 12

Ingredients:

For the Base:

- 9 Medjool dates, pitted
- 1/3 cup Brazil nuts
- 2 tablespoons maple syrup
- 1/3 cup walnuts
- 2 tablespoons water
- 3 tablespoons cacao powder

For the Chocolate Cheesecake:

- 1/2 cup cacao powder
- 1 1/2 cups cashews, soaked for 10 minutes in warm water, drained
- 1/3 cup liquid coconut oil
- 1 teaspoon vanilla extract, unsweetened
- 1/3 cup maple syrup

- 1/3 cup water

For the Orange Cheesecake:

- 2 oranges, juiced
- 1/4 cup maple syrup
- 1 cup cashews, soaked for 10 minutes in warm water, drained
- 1 teaspoon vanilla extract, unsweetened
- 2 tablespoons coconut butter
- 1/2 cup liquid coconut oil
- 2 oranges, zested
- 4 drops of orange essential oil

For the Chocolate Topping:

- 3 tablespoons cacao powder
- 3 drops of orange essential oil
- 2 tablespoons liquid coconut oil
- 3 tablespoons maple syrup

Directions:

1. Prepare the base, and for this, place all its ingredients in a food processor and pulse for 3 to 5 minutes until the thick paste comes together.

2. Take a cake tin, place crust mixture in it and spread and press the mixture evenly in the bottom, and freeze until required.
3. Prepare the chocolate cheesecake, and for this, place all its ingredients in a food processor and pulse for 2 minutes until smooth.
4. Pour the chocolate cheesecake mixture on top of the prepared base, smooth the top and freeze for 20 minutes until set.
5. Then prepare the orange cheesecake and for this, place all its ingredients in a food processor, and pulse for 2 minutes until smooth
6. Top orange cheesecake mixture over chocolate cheesecake, and then freeze for 3 hours until hardened.
7. Then prepare the chocolate topping and for this, take a bowl, add all the ingredients in it and stir until well combined.
8. Spread chocolate topping over the top, freeze the cake for 10 minutes until the topping has hardened and then slice to serve.

Nutrition:
- Calories: 508 Cal

- Fat: 34.4 g
- Carbs: 44 g
- Protein: 8 g
- Fiber: 3 g

Coconut Ice Cream Cheesecake

Preparation Time: 3 hours

Cooking Time: 0 minute

Servings: 4

Ingredients:

For the First Layer:

1 cup mixed nuts

3/4 cup dates, soaked for 10 minutes in warm water

2 tablespoons almond milk

For the Second Layer:

1 medium avocado, diced

1 cup cashew nuts, soaked for 10 minutes in warm water

3 cups strawberries, sliced

1 tablespoon chia seeds, soaked in 3 tablespoons soy milk

1/2 cup agave

1 cup melted coconut oil

1/2 cup shredded coconut

1 lime, juiced

Directions:

1. Prepare the first layer, and for this, place all its ingredients in a food processor and pulse for 3 to 5 minutes until the thick paste comes together.
2. Take a springform pan, place crust mixture in it and spread and press the mixture evenly in the bottom, and freeze until required.
3. Prepare the second layer, and for this, place all its ingredients in a food processor and pulse for 2 minutes until smooth.
4. Pour the second layer on top of the first layer, smooth the top, and freeze for 4 hours until hard.
5. Serve straight away.

Nutrition:

- Calories: 411.3 Cal
- Fat: 30.8 g
- Carbs: 28.7 g
- Protein: 4.7 g
- Fiber: 1.3 g

Matcha Coconut Cream Pie

Preparation Time: 5 minutes

Cooking Time: 0 minute

Servings: 4

Ingredients:

For the Crust:

  1/2 cup ground flaxseed

  3/4 cup shredded dried coconut

  1 cup Medjool dates, pitted

  3/4 cup dehydrated buckwheat groats

  1/4 teaspoons sea salt

For the Filling:

  1 cup dried coconut flakes

  4 cups of coconut meat

  1/4 cup and 2 Tablespoons coconut nectar

  1/2 Tablespoons vanilla extract, unsweetened

  1/4 teaspoons sea salt

  2/3 cup and 2 Tablespoons coconut butter

  1 Tablespoons matcha powder

  1/2 cup coconut water

Directions:

Prepare the crust, and for this, place all its ingredients in a food processor and pulse for 3 to 5 minutes until the thick paste comes together.

Take a 6-inch springform pan, grease it with oil, place crust mixture in it and spread and press the mixture evenly in the bottom and along the sides, and freeze until required.

Prepare the filling and for this, place all its ingredients in a food processor, and pulse for 2 minutes until smooth.

Pour the filling into prepared pan, smooth the top, and freeze for 4 hours until set.

Cut pie into slices and then serve

Nutrition:

- Calories: 209 Cal
- Fat: 18 g
- Carbs: 10 g
- Protein: 1 g
- Fiber: 2 g

Chocolate Peanut Butter Cake

Preparation Time: 5 minutes

Cooking Time: 0 minute

Servings: 8

Ingredients:

For the Base:

- 1 tablespoon ground flaxseeds
- 1/8 cup millet
- 3/4 cup peanuts
- 1/4 cup and 2 tablespoons shredded coconut unsweetened
- 1 teaspoon hemp oil
- 1/2 cup flake oats

For the Date Layer:

- 1 tablespoon ground flaxseed
- 1 cup dates
- 1 tablespoon hemp hearts
- 2 tablespoons coconut
- 3 tablespoons cacao

For the Chocolate Layer:

- 3/4 cup coconut flour
- 2 tablespoons and 2 teaspoons cacao
- 1 tablespoon maple syrup
- 8 tablespoons warm water
- 2 tablespoons coconut oil
- 1/2 cup coconut milk
- 2 tablespoons ground flaxseed

For the Chocolate Topping:

- 7 ounces coconut cream
- 2 1/2 tablespoons cacao
- 1 teaspoon agave
- For Assembly:
- 1/2 cup almond butter

Directions:

1. Prepare the crust, and for this, place all its ingredients in a food processor and pulse for 3 to 5 minutes until the thick paste comes together.
2. Take a loaf tin, grease it with oil, place crust mixture in it and spread and press the mixture evenly in the bottom and along the sides, and freeze until required.

3. Prepare the date layer, and for this, place all its ingredients in a food processor and pulse for 2 minutes until smooth.
4. Prepare the chocolate layer, and for this, place flour and flax in a bowl and stir until combined.
5. Take a saucepan, add remaining ingredients, stir until mixed and cook for 5 minutes until melted and smooth.
6. Add it into the flour mixture, stir until dough comes together, and set aside.
7. Prepare the chocolate topping, place all its ingredients in a food processor and pulse for 3 to 5 minutes until smooth.
8. Press date layer into the base layer, refrigerate for 1 hour, then press chocolate layer on its top, finish with chocolate topping, refrigerate for 3 hours and serve.

Nutrition:
- Calories: 390 Cal
- Fat: 24.3 g
- Carbs: 35 g
- Protein: 10.3 g
- Fiber: 2 g

Chocolate Raspberry Brownies

Preparation Time: 4 hours

Cooking Time: 0 minute

Servings: 4

Ingredients:

For the Chocolate Brownie Base:

12 Medjool Dates, pitted

3/4 cup oat flour

3/4 cup almond meal

3 tablespoons cacao

1 teaspoon vanilla extract, unsweetened

1/8 teaspoon sea salt

3 tablespoons water

1/2 cup pecans, chopped

For the Raspberry Cheesecake:

3/4 cup cashews, soaked, drained

6 tablespoons agave nectar

1/2 cup raspberries

1 teaspoon vanilla extract, unsweetened

1 lemon, juiced

6 tablespoons liquid coconut oil

For the Chocolate Coating:

2 1/2 tablespoons cacao powder

3 3/4 tablespoons coconut Oil

2 tablespoons maple syrup

1/8 teaspoon sea salt

Directions:

Prepare the crust, and for this, place all its ingredients in a food processor and pulse for 3 to 5 minutes until the thick paste comes together.

Take a 6-inch springform pan, grease it with oil, place crust mixture in it and spread and press the mixture evenly in the bottom and along the sides, and freeze until required.

Prepare the cheesecake topping, and for this, place all its ingredients in a food processor and pulse for 2 minutes until smooth.

Pour the filling into prepared pan, smooth the top, and freeze for 8 hours until solid.

Prepare the chocolate coating and for this, whisk together all its ingredients until smooth, drizzle on top of the cake and then serve.

Nutrition:

Calories: 371 Cal

Fat: 42.4 g

Carbs: 42 g

Protein: 5.5 g

Fiber: 2 g

Brownie Batter

Preparation Time: 5 minutes

Cooking Time: 0 minute

Servings: 4

Ingredients:

4 Medjool dates, pitted, soaked in warm water

1.5 ounces chocolate, unsweetened, melted

2 tablespoons maple syrup

4 tablespoons tahini

½ teaspoon vanilla extract, unsweetened

1 tablespoon cocoa powder, unsweetened

1/8 teaspoon sea salt

1/8 teaspoon espresso powder

2 to 4 tablespoons almond milk, unsweetened

Directions:

Place all the ingredients in a food processor and process for 2 minutes until combined.

Set aside until required.

Nutrition:

Calories: 44 Cal

Fat: 1 g

Carbs: 6 g

Protein: 2 g

Fiber: 0 g

Strawberry Mousse

Preparation Time: 5 minutes

Cooking Time: 15 minutes

Servings: 4

Ingredients:

- 8 ounces coconut milk, unsweetened
- 2 tablespoons honey
- 5 strawberries

Directions:

1. Place berries in a blender and pulse until the smooth mixture comes together.
2. Place milk in a bowl, whisk until whipped, and then add remaining ingredients and stir until combined.
3. Refrigerate the mousse for 10 minutes and then serve.

Nutrition:

Calories: 145 Cal

Fat: 23 g

Carbs: 15 g

Protein: 5 g

Fiber: 1 g

Blueberry Mousse

Preparation Time: 20 minutes

Cooking Time: 0 minute

Servings: 2

Ingredients:

1 cup wild blueberries

1 cup cashews, soaked for 10 minutes, drained

1/2 teaspoon berry powder

2 tablespoons coconut oil, melted

1 tablespoon lemon juice

1 teaspoon vanilla extract, unsweetened

1/4 cup hot water

Directions:

Place all the ingredients in a food processor and process for 2 minutes until smooth.

Set aside until required.

Nutrition:

Calories: 433 Cal

Fat: 32.3 g

Carbs: 44 g

Protein: 5.1 g

Tips To Keep Motivated

Staying motivated on an exercise plan can be tough. You might start out with all of the best intentions, but after a few weeks or so, you will get worn out and not want to continue. It is much easier to just sit on the couch and hope that everything works out the way that you would like. While you know all of the great reasons to get up and do some exercising, it just is not as much fun, or at least is more work, than some of the other things you might want to do. Here are some of the best tips that you can use that will help you to keep motivated and get in a great workout every day.

Set some goals

Before you even head out to the gym, make sure that you are setting some goals. Make them challenging enough that you will need to put in some work, but simple enough that you would actually be able to get them done if you work hard. For example, it is not a good idea to say you will lose ten pounds a week, but saying you want to lose 2 pounds is reasonable.

Write down these goals from the beginning. They can be anything that you want as long as they give you a bit of a challenge and make you work for it. You can say that you will lose a certain amount of weight over time, go by the measurements in your body, or you can even choose to go for a specific amount of time or reps. It is up to you, just make sure that you are having some fun and working hard while at the gym.

Bring along music

Getting on the treadmill and staring at a wall for 30 to 60 minutes is going to get boring fast. You might enjoy it the first few times, but after that, the activity is not going to be as much fun and you will find that your motivation starts to slip away. This is why you should consider bringing something along to do while you are working out. This can be almost anything. Many people like to bring along some of their favorite music. This allows them to have something fun and upbeat to listen to while they are working out plus can get them pumped up and in the right mood to keep going.

Do an activity you love

It honestly does not matter how much you think an activity is going to help you to lose weight, if you are not enjoying it, you are less likely to keep up with it and you are not going to lose weight. Find something that you like doing, such as biking, swimming, weight lifting, walking, running, or maybe even a group class, and then do that. Even if it is not burning as many calories as another activity, at least you are having fun. The more fun you have with an activity, the better results you will have because you are more likely to keep going with it.

Try a new activity

It is always good to mix things up when you are at the gym. Even if you love an activity, you might find that after a few months of doing it all of the time, you are getting bored with it. Plus, your body is going to become used to a certain activity and you will not get the same results if you keep doing it. Find a few activities that you enjoy, or try a few new ones, and the switch them around on occasion. This allows you to do something new, continue having fun, and you can continue seeing results all at the same time.

Find a friend

For some people, the way that they get some motivation is to find a friend who is going to work out with them. This person should be someone who is looking for the same goals and who will be able to hold you accountable to show up. When you are doing the work outs on your own, it is easy to say that you'll get to it tomorrow and then you never go back. On the other hand, when you know that someone is waiting at the gym for you, you might feel a bit more obligated to show up. Once there, you might as well get in a good work out since you went to all of the trouble. This means you get in a work out much more often than you would on your own, and the results will be much better.

Get outside

You do not need to spend all of your time inside in the gym. When the weather is nice and you are having some trouble getting to the gym, why not take a good walk outside. This is one of the best ways to get in a good workout and can help to lift up your mood because you are getting plenty of fresh air and sunlight.

Reward yourself

Whenever you are able to reach some of your goals while working out, you should take the time to reward yourself. This allows you to feel good about the hard work you are doing and even gives you something to look forward to. You should not let the award be about food since you are trying to lose weight and this can ruin your plans. But choosing to go out a night with friends, go see a movie, purchase some new clothes, or give yourself a spa day can be great incentives to keep yourself going.

Each person is going to have some of their own methods to use that will motivate them to see success. While it might be hard to get on a good workout program, it is important to find a way to get on one and stick with it for your overall health. Once you get started and do it well for a few weeks, it becomes a routine and is much easier to do. Follow some of the tips in this and see how easy it can be to get in your required work out each day.

Don't Forget To Exercise

There are several things that you can do in order to meet your weight loss goals. These include cutting back on the number of calories that you eat each day and starting a healthy exercise program are two great ways to meet your goals, especially if you combine them both together. It is still important to maintain an exercise program even after you have reached your weight loss goals in order to maintain the weight loss. After you have decided to go on a diet and start an exercise program the first thing that you will be asking yourself is how much exercise that you will need.

An important step that you should consider doing before you start any exercise plan is to talk to your doctor. They will be able to tell you if the plan is good for you, how much exercise you should do, and give you any advice and suggestions about what will work in your situation. They will also be able to do a complete checkup in order to make sure that they are no underlying problems in your health that could affect what types of exercises you are able to do.

You should consider some basic considerations when

you start a diet. It is important to remember that there are no magic pills or amazing diet plans that will help you to lose the weigh overnight. Even if you do lose a lot of weight quickly on a particular plan, it is not

There are no magic exercise plans that work for everyone and help everyone to lose the weight. Each person has a different body and responds in different ways to certain types of exercise. It might take some trial and error in order to find out which exercises that you enjoy and which ones work the best for you.

If you are looking to exercise to lose weight there are some guidelines that you should follow. It is recommended by the Centers for Disease Control and Prevention that you try to get at least two hours and 30 minutes of exercise in a week in order to lose weight. This might sound like a lot but it ends up only being about 30 minutes five days a week; of course, the more exercise that you do, the greater the results of the weight loss. You will have to incorporate more exercise into your routine if you do not plan to cut back on your calories in order to see weight loss.

Some activities that you should include in your exercise plan include cardiovascular exercises such as walking, running, biking, hiking and swimming. In order to burn the largest amount of calories during your workout you need to elevate your heart rate and keep it at that rate for an extended time during the workout.

It is not a good idea to spend all of your time concentrating on aerobic exercises. While they are great for your heart and in helping you to burn calories and lose weight, you should include also other activities in your work out. These include strength training and stretching exercises, which can help make your bones and muscles stronger and help slim your waistline.

You can get just so many benefits from exercising. One of the benefits includes weight loss. Just for spending an hour doing a low impact exercise a 160 pound person can lose somewhere around 350 calories. If you decide to do a higher impact activity such as running you could lose up to 900 calories in that hour, which is way more than you need to burn in order to lose a pound per week.

Just how much exercise that you need in your exercise program will depend on how much weight you will want to lose? If you live a very sedentary life, and you want to lose a lot of weight, you will have to include more exercise in your day than someone who has a job that keeps them moving all day. It is a good idea to start with 30 minutes a couple of times a day and slowly build up to working out between 30-60 minutes at least five days a week.

The Benefits of Exercising

Weight Loss

The first reason why many people will choose to exercise and work out is because they are looking to lose weight. Every weight loss and diet plan in the world will spell out how important it is to get in a good exercise program if you really want to lose weight. While limiting your calories can help out a lot, you are only able to limit those so much and exercising can help pick up the slack so that you are able to lose more. Pick a moderate to high intensity work out for the best results.

Heart Health

For you to really get a good workout, you will need to get that heart pumping and working hard. When the heart is functioning at this level, it is becoming stronger than ever before. When you sit on the couch, the heart barely has to move in order to get the nutrients all around the body so it is not becoming very strong. With a good work out that makes you sweat and gets the heart up a bit, you can work on its strength and become stronger in no time.

Brain Functioning

Studies have shown that getting in some exercise during the week is critical if you want your brain to function the way that it is supposed to. Exercise can help increase the flow of oxygen and blood to the brain which opens it up for working so much more efficiently. An added bonus is that exercise can help you out with your memory. This is important for those who are aging and need a bit of help recalling important events and facts. Of course, you may be able to find a lot of benefits of this as a younger person as well when you exercise right before a test and are better able to recall the facts you learn.

Stress

Stress is a daily part of life for most people and there is not much that they can do in order to get it to go away. But there are some things that you can do to reduce the amount of stress that you are feeling and to get yourself to look and feel better about the stress. Any time that the stress is starting to get too much for you, go and do a quick run or pop in your favorite work out movie. This will allow you to take a break from the stress you are feeling and you can better get back on track with other things.

Cholesterol

High cholesterol is a huge problem that a lot of people are dealing with because of the high fat diet found in this country. When you get on a good workout program, you can help to reduce the amount of bad cholesterol that is in the blood while also increasing the kind of good that is there.

Blood Pressure

When eating a diet that is high in sodium, or when you sit on the couch all day and do not perform some kind of physical activity, it is easy for you to get high blood pressure. One of the first things that the doctor is going to recommend that you do is get out and start exercising at least five days a week. This will allow the heart to function properly, your cholesterol to go lower, and your body to be better able to reduce the salts that are in there. All of this combines to allow your blood pressure to go way down.

Diabetes

Even the symptoms of diabetes can be controlled better when you are on a good exercise program. You will find that the body is able to metabolize the sugars that you are consuming much better when you are on this kind of program. Plus you are less likely to crave unhealthy and sugary foods so your insulin will not be under as much stress. If you are suffering from diabetes or pre-diabetes, it is best if you are able to get on a good workout program as soon as possible.

Mood

Your mood can be influenced by how much you exercise. Those who are depressed and down a lot of the time are the ones who rarely if ever get out there and do a good work out. Think about it this way, the few times that you have been to the gym and got in a really good workout how did you feel? Most people will say they felt good and that they were happy and on a little cloud for the rest of the day. Well, if you get on a good exercise program, you will be able to feel this way all of the time. Overall your mood will begin to improve. If you have depression, you may be able to cure it with a good exercise program. Even if you are not suffering from a mood disorder, you can benefit from the mood enhancement that comes from a good work out program.

Digestion

For many of those who are suffering from issues with their digestive tracts, a good work out program is able to help out with this. You should get in at least five days of moderate activity for 30 minutes on each day in order to see some of these great benefits on your digestive system in no time.

Self-confidence

For many, the way that they look and feel can determine how confident they are in themselves. When they start out on an exercise program and begin to lose weight, plus get all of the great health benefits that are listed above, they are going to feel a little bit better and you will notice a huge surge in the amount of self-confidence that they are feeling. They will begin to like the way that they look and will want to show it off. Just a few minutes of exercise each day can make this into a reality.

Intermittent Fasting Strategy With No Meat Diet

Fasting is not a new thing, as it has been practiced through the ages for different reasons. People fast for religious, spiritual, medical, and cultural reasons. People even fast in protest of something like the cutting down of trees in the rainforest, or the neglect of human rights.

However, in recent years scientists have become more interested in the health benefits of fasting. There are long and short-term benefits of intermittent fasting, especially when a person follows a plant-based whole-foods diet.

Some of the health benefits of intermittent fasting on a plant-based diet may include:

Age benefits — it may prolong a person's life and may have anti-aging benefits.

Weight loss — it may help with weight loss when done in a properly controlled environment.

Sleep — it is thought the intermittent fasting helps to

regulate the circadian rhythm. The circadian rhythm is what determines the body's sleep patterns. When this rhythm is regulated, a person falls asleep a lot easier and has a better quality of sleep. A better quality of sleep means a person wakes up feeling refreshed.

Lowers the risk of disease — intermittent fasting may help to increase insulin sensitivity, prevent cancer, increase cell turnover (autophagy), lower blood pressure and cholesterol.

Brain function — intermittent fasting is thought to be able to boot brain function to increase a person's concentration and improve their mental acuity.

When we eat, our body's insulin level rises in order to store away excess energy by either:

Breaking carbohydrates into glucose to be stored in the liver of muscle.

Once the liver has reached its limit of glucose, it gets turned into fat.

This basically means that fat that cannot be stored in the liver is then taken and stored in fat deposits around the body.

When we do not eat, our bodies basically reverse the process as the insulin level will drop and the body starts to burn the stored fat for energy.

How intermittent fasting helps is to stop the body from being in the "fed" state all the time, to not being fed state. When the body is not being fed and is in a hunger state, the body starts to use up all the excess fat. Intermittent fasting helps to maintain the body's balance and clean out its pantry of stored fat (glucose). There is no actual set time limit to fast or not to fast; you can fast from 16 hours to a few days. Although if you are thinking of fasting for a few days it is advisable to do it under strict medical supervision.

You can also fast for a day, from 7 am to 6 pm. Intermittent fasting diet is usually split into the following patterns:

Fasting hours

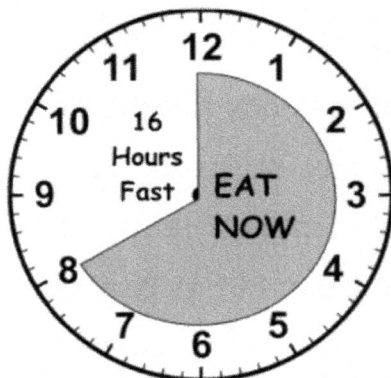

Fasting should be done within strict daily time windows. 16-hours of intermittent fasting and 8-hours of eating. This means you have to spend 16 hours of the day not eating; you then have an 8-hour window in which to eat. It does not mean to gorge yourself for 8 hours, though. It means to eat at regular intervals, following a controlled number of calories. This is a good pattern for beginners to start with.

20-hours of intermittent fasting and 4-hours of eating. This intermittent fasting is for more advanced intermittent fasting. It requires 20 hrs of fasting with only a 4-hour eating window.

24-hour fasting should be done on one day and then the day has one meal. The day two meals, and so on.

Fasting Days

ALTERNATE-DAY FASTING

DAY 1	DAY 2	DAY 3	DAY 4	DAY 5	DAY 6	DAY 7
Eats normally	24-hour fast OR Eat only a few hundred calories	Eats normally	24-hour fast OR Eat only a few hundred calories	Eats normally	24-hour fast OR Eat only a few hundred calories	Eats normally

Daily fasting time windows should only be a day, within or for a certain period of days.

5 days off intermittent fasting and 2 days of intermittent fasting is the version that has the most medical support. This is the version of intermittent fasting a doctor may recommend if you are under medical supervision or have sought medical advice. You spend 5 days eating regularly, on a plant-based diet and 2 days of fasting following one of the time windows in the above. It should also be noted that during these

time windows of the 2 days fasting, a person should only eat around 500 calories per day.

1 day off 1 day for a week is where you would have one day of regular eating and one day of fasting. Once again, on the days of fasting, eating time windows only permit up to 500 calories a day.

Extended fasting is not recommended unless under strict medical supervision.

There are many things to consider before you attempt intermittent fasting, especially if you are going to continue exercising or have any health conditions. But when done properly with a plant-based diet, intermittent fasting can offer a person a lot of health and weight loss benefits.

Conclusion

I hope that by this point in the, you are convinced that as a vegan, you can consume the proper foods to achieve the nutrients that you need to thrive. There are going to be many doubters out there in the world—do not let them convince you that your diet is wrong. You are the only person you need to convince that a vegan diet is the best option for you.

You have made the decision to not only better your health but also make the world around you better. At this point, you are saving animals and helping the environment. Your diet choices are beneficial to you and the world around you. Now, you know just how delicious your diet can be. While some look at a vegan diet as restrictive, you know better. As a vegan, you get to have your cake and eat it as well!

As you can see, it is possible to lead an athlete life also for those who choose the vegan lifestyle.

Rather, in many respects this is a choice to be recommended given that it has many advantages (not only from a muscle and training perspective) without any obstacle concerning the required protein intake from those who play sports–even those that are very demanding or require excessive efforts.

The important thing is to always out what the needs of our organism are in order to create solid foundations on which to build and shape our body.

Using different recipes and varying the diet are great help, not only to supply our body with the necessary nutrients, but also to make more enjoyable an act that needs to be repeated often throughout the day.

As you become more comfortable with the recipes provided in this, I invite you to add some ideas of your own! The best part of a vegan diet is how versatile it can be. If you have favorite vegetables, throw them in! There is no one way to cook—make it your own and enjoy your diet every single day. I wish you the best of luck on your vegan journey. Now, let's get cooking!